I0438291

Baring Your Breast

Mammograms: A Positive Experience

by
Carole Aydell, R.T. (R) (M)

Edited by Tara Mullee

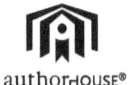

authorHOUSE®

AuthorHouse™
1663 Liberty Drive, Suite 200
Bloomington, IN 47403
www.authorhouse.com
Phone: 1-800-839-8640

This book is a work of non-fiction. Unless otherwise noted, the author
and the publisher make no explicit guarantees as to the accuracy of
the information contained in this book and in some cases, names
of people and places have been altered to protect their privacy.

First published by AuthorHouse 2/11/2008

ISBN: 978-1-4343-4816-6 (e)
ISBN: 978-1-4343-4880-7 (sc)

Library of Congress Control Number: 2007908672

Printed in the United States of America
Bloomington, Indiana

This book is printed on acid-free paper.

The information in this book is not intended in any way to be a substitute for the expertise, judgment, and diagnoses of qualified health care professionals. The author specifically disclaims any responsibility for any liability, loss, or risk, personal or otherwise, which is incurred as a consequence, directly or indirectly, by the use and application of the contents of this book.

Daddy, I miss you every day.

Contents

Dedication

This book is dedicated to the memory of Alicia, who died of breast cancer in 1987. She was 27.

Her beautiful spirit will always be remembered.

Alicia and I were friends and cheerleaders at our high school in French Settlement, Louisiana. I was in my first year of radiology school when she died, and when I graduated the next year, performing mammograms was the last job most technologists wanted to do. Although mammograms had been performed for many years, the practice was still intimidating, and many technologists just did not want any part of it. I, however, entered mammography right after graduation and discovered that radiology school had failed to prepare me for the number of women with only one breast—or none at all—due to mastectomies. Compared with today, that number was very high, and those were just the women who survived. Unfortunately, Alicia was not one of them.

One organization that exists today to help people like Alicia is the Young Survival Coalition, which works with researchers and doctors to educate young women, medical professionals, caregivers, and the general public about breast cancer. It also provides a forum for young women with breast cancer to discuss vital issues by hosting survivor-education programs and co-sponsoring international conferences on this topic.

While most breast cancers occur in women older than 40, younger women can and do get breast cancer. According to the Young Survival Coalition, more than 250,000 U.S. women 40 and younger are living with breast cancer, and 11,500 will be diagnosed in the next year. In fact, the YSC states that breast cancer is the leading cause of cancer-related deaths in girls as young as 15.

No effective breast-cancer screening tools exist for women younger than 35, which makes it imperative that these women perform monthly breast self-exams, have yearly clinical exams and, if they find a lump, have ultrasounds and/or biopsies.

For information on how to support the YSC, log on to www.youngsurvival.org, e-mail info@youngsurvival.org, or call (212) 206-6610 or (877) YSC-1011.

Part of the proceeds from this book will go to supporting YSC.

Introduction

Over the years, my patients have encouraged me to write a book that would change women's negative attitudes toward mammograms.

So many women misunderstand this life-saving process. My book is for all you who have had extremely painful mammograms and for all the women who are afraid of having their first one. This is not a procedure you should fear. We, as women, should be appreciative that we have the technology today to detect breast cancer at such an early stage.

After you're finished reading, I hope you'll have a better understanding of four interrelated issues: Why mammograms should not be painful and what to do about it if they are; the importance of breast self-exams; how we can drastically reduce the number of women we lose each year to breast cancer; and why early detection is your only protection.

By sharing this information with you, I hope you will realize you are not alone in your fear of mammograms. Learning about the mammogram process will help eliminate your fear and show you that it's a simple procedure that has suffered from a bad reputation.

The National Cancer Institute says one in eight women will develop breast cancer in her lifetime. More than 40,000 women will die of the disease this year in the United States alone. It is second only to lung cancer as the leading cause of cancer deaths in American women.

You should encourage, not discourage, those you care about to get yearly mammograms and clinical exams, and to perform breast self-exams every month. By spreading the word to friends, co-workers, mothers, daughters, and sisters—and even men, who are also at risk for the disease— you can help save their lives.

Patient's Story

"It's breast cancer."

That's all I heard. Everything the doctor said after those three words—"We'll aggressively treat this disease," and "If we had found it sooner …"—I heard none of it.

"It's breast cancer."

I could not hear or think of anything else. The words loomed before me. "It can't be," I kept repeating to myself. "It must be a mistake. I don't smoke or drink. I wear sunscreen, watch my diet, exercise regularly. No one in my family has breast cancer. This just can't be happening to me."

I don't remember the doctor leaving the room; all I could see was the paper cup of water in front of me. I reached for it, my hands shaking. I took the cup of water, still in shock over the reason I was there—the reason I received the call from the nurse telling me I needed to come in to discuss my biopsy results.

Those three little words.

"It's breast cancer."

1. No More Excuses

"I don't have any family history of breast cancer."

Don't Fear It. Find It.

People are afraid of the unknown. The same is true for women and mammograms. Even though about one in eight will be diagnosed with breast cancer, many women still refuse to get mammograms. They are afraid it will hurt or that the mammogram will reveal breast cancer, which is an issue they don't want to confront or deal with—the "ignorance is bliss" mentality. But with breast cancer, ignorance is not bliss. Ignorance could be death.

"I've been too busy," some women say to explain why they don't get mammograms—too busy working, raising children, taking care of sick parents or relatives. So you haven't had a mammogram in years, or you've never had one, because you've been busy with daily life or with helping others. But what about yourself? Do you think breast cancer will wait until you have more free time? Do you think breast cancer waits for anybody?

Some women think that because there's no history of breast cancer in their families they have no chance of getting it. This is a false assumption. Although you are at higher risk if your mother, sister, daughter, or maternal grandmother has been diagnosed with it, all women have some risk of breast cancer and most women with the disease do not have any family history. Men can also develop breast cancer, although it is not as common.

Let's take a quick look at the numbers. The National Cancer Institute estimates that 40,460 women and 450 men will die from breast cancer in the United States in 2007. In fact, women living in North America have the highest rate of breast cancer in the world.

Despite these frightening statistics, quite a few women think it's not necessary to get a mammogram unless their doctors explicitly tell them to do so. Wrong. First of all, you do not have to make a doctor's appointment to get a mammogram. Some mammogram facilities do not require a prescription if you are older than 35. If they do, you can simply call your doctor's office and have an order faxed to the facility you wish to visit. Second, if you have a doctor's appointment but your doctor does not mention mammograms, then be sure to ask him or her about it.

Sadly, many women think they are unable to get mammograms because they don't have health insurance. However, certain places administer them for free. Call the American Cancer Society anytime at 1-800-ACS-2345 to get a list of facilities in your area that offer free mammograms, ultrasounds and biopsies. Also, some facilities offer cash discounts or payment plans for people who don't have insurance. If you don't know which clinics in your area offer these options, simply call around and ask. A few phone calls are a small price to pay for a checkup that could save your life. Remember, the longer you let your cancer go undetected, the more extensive—and expensive— the treatment. Women who ignore the health of their breasts face larger, more dangerous, and less treatable tumors than women who keep a sharp eye out for breast cancer. The earlier the diagnosis, the better your prognosis. It's up to you.

More than one patient has told me that even though her mother had breast cancer, her sister refuses to get mammograms, because she "just doesn't want to know." Again, the "ignorance is bliss" theory. Let me reiterate: BREAST CANCER IS CURABLE IF YOU CATCH IT EARLY ENOUGH. How are you going to catch it in the early stages if you're not looking for it, not doing your breast self-exams every month, not getting a physical exam by a professional and a mammogram every year after your 40th birthday?

Nobody wants breast cancer. But if it's there, you do want to find it.

Give Mammograms a Chance.

In addition to the fear of being diagnosed with cancer, many women are also afraid of the mammogram itself. Some may have had painful mammogram experiences, and others have heard horror stories about the procedure.

Early in my career, one of my patients, a woman in her 60s, hadn't had a mammogram in eight years. When I asked her why, her response shocked me.

"After the last mammogram I had, I swore I'd never have another one."

She was the first patient to say that to me, but since then I've heard the same answer from countless other women. One of the reasons I'm writing this book is to reach out to those of you who feel this way, those of you who had a painful mammogram once and don't want to go through it again. I don't blame you. No one wants to get hurt. But guess what? Mammograms do not have to be painful.

One of my patients actually cried as she asked me, "Does it really hurt as badly as they say?" She told me she had heard so many horrible stories about having a mammogram that she kept putting it off until her sister was diagnosed with breast cancer.

"It's a shame it took your sister having breast cancer to get you in," I told her. "No, I'm not going to hurt you. The procedure was never designed to hurt anyone. It's awkward, yes, because we have one machine that fits all and no two women are alike. But let me show you, and then you can tell me how bad it was."

After the mammogram, my initially terrified patient said she couldn't believe it was so easy. "The pressure felt tight," she said, "but it didn't hurt."

Another patient once told me that ever since she told her female co-workers she was going in for her first mammogram, they had barraged her with "jokes."

"They told me you're going to flatten me like a pancake," she said. "I got three e-mails in the last two weeks, one about preparing yourself for a mammogram by slamming your breast in a refrigerator door or by lying on the garage floor and letting a car roll over your breast. I couldn't sleep thinking about this."

After her mammogram, she also was amazed at how painless it was.

What input do you contribute at your workplace or among your friends when someone says she's going in for her first mammogram? Instead of sending "funny" e-mails to women who are about to get a mammogram, give them this book to read. Even if you've had a bad experience with mammograms, don't scare other women into thinking all mammograms must be terrible ordeals. Remember that mammograms were not designed to be painful. If you did have a bad experience, you owe it to yourself and to the people who care about you to give mammograms a second chance.

In this book, you'll learn why your first mammogram may have been painful and ways to make sure your next one is more comfortable. Mammograms have come a long way since they were first introduced as a screening device for breast cancer. Every year, manufacturers strive to improve the quality and performance of the machines. The film manufacturers have developed mammogram film so sensitive it requires a special processor to develop it. There are even machines designed to "read" your mammogram before the radiologist reads it, thereby giving your mammogram two readings. The technologists who perform mammograms now are required to undergo additional training to become skilled, certified mammographers.

So what should you expect when you give mammograms a second chance, or when you get your first mammogram? The next two chapters will explain the types of mammograms available, how the process works, and how to ensure your experience is a good one.

2. Types of Mammograms

"I kept putting off having a mammogram until my sister was diagnosed with breast cancer."

What Is a Mammogram?

For those of you who are completely new to this, an analog mammogram is a low-dose X-ray of the breast. Pictures, also called images or exposures, are taken during the mammogram and exposed to film. The film that is developed from the X-ray exposures can show both malignant (cancerous) and benign (non-cancerous) tumors in your breast, just like regular X-rays show the bones inside your body.

Digital mammography uses computer image processing. This state-of-the-art technology greatly reduces the amount of radiation exposure the patient receives, and it gives the radiologist more tools with which to adjust the contrast of the image without additional exposure to the patient.

According to the American Cancer Society, mammography can detect about 90 percent of breast cancers found in women without symptoms. That makes mammography the most effective method of early detection, because it can identify the disease in precancerous stages before the actual cancer develops. These precancerous cells can usually be removed with a biopsy.

One reason why mammography doesn't catch the other 10 percent of breast cancers is breast density. Today, digital mammography has greatly improved the quality of images, especially those of dense breasts. Younger women who haven't had children or hormone replacement therapy generally have denser breasts, which are harder to penetrate with X-rays. Mammography is, therefore, usually more accurate with older, postmenopausal women. However, mammography is still an indispensable tool for all women.

Mammograms may also miss a small percentage of breast cancers due to a faster growth rate of the tumor. The mammogram could also fail to see the small, early signs of an abnormality because of the location of the tumor or other factors. This makes your self-exams and clinical exams all the more important. You can feel some lumps before they are detected by a mammogram. By using all three tools—mammography, breast self-exams and clinical breast exams—you increase your chance of discovering the cancer early.

Screening Mammograms

When you go to the mammography facility, you will receive either a screening or diagnostic mammogram, depending on your medical needs.

A screening mammogram is equivalent to a checkup. It's a screening of your breasts that is not prompted by any abnormal symptoms. It should be done every other year starting at age 35 and then once a year after age 40. However, if you have a family history of breast cancer or other high-risk factors, you may have to begin getting yearly mammograms at age 35 or even 30. Don't be shy about alerting your doctor to these risk factors so you can discuss these issues together.

The most significant risk factor for having breast cancer is simply being female. But remember that men can also develop the disease.

According to the National Cancer Institute, other risk factors include but are not limited to:

- Your age. The older you are, the greater your risk.

- Personal history. If you've been diagnosed with another kind of cancer, you have an increased risk of developing breast cancer. Also, a woman who has had breast cancer in one breast has an increased risk of getting the disease in her other breast.

- Family history. A woman's risk is higher if her mother, sister, daughter, or maternal grandmother had breast cancer. This may also apply to women with other relatives, on either her mother's or her father's side of the family, who had breast cancer.

- Certain breast changes. Some women's breasts contain cells that look abnormal under a microscope. Certain breast abnormalities, such as atypical hyperplasia, a benign condition in which the number of cells increases abnormally, are markers for potential breast cancer.

- Reproductive history. Having your first child after age 30, or having no children at all, increases your risk of developing breast cancer. Research suggests that having an abortion or a miscarriage does not increase your risk.

- Menstrual history. Women who had their first menstrual period early and went through menopause late are at increased risk.

- Obesity, especially after menopause. Some studies show that gaining weight after menopause increases the risk of breast cancer.

- Lack of physical activity.

- Recent use of oral contraceptives (birth-control pills) or postmenopausal estrogen. Women who take menopausal hormone therapy with estrogen plus progestin after menopause appear to be at a higher risk for breast cancer. Women who took diethylstilbestrol (DES), a synthetic form of estrogen that was given to some pregnant women in the United States between 1940 and 1971, have a slightly increased risk of the disease. Researchers are studying the effects, if any, of DES on these women's daughters.

- The use of tobacco products, which lowers the body's immune system and makes it less able to defend itself against disease. Smokers are at an increased risk of breast cancer and all cancers, especially lung cancer—which kills even more women every year than breast cancer does. The more cigarettes a woman smokes per day, the higher her risk, but any amount, no matter how small, is dangerous.

- Alcoholic beverages. Some studies suggest a link between the amount of alcohol a woman drinks and her risk of breast cancer.

Diet is another potential risk factor being studied today. Some evidence suggests that a low-fat diet rich in fruits and vegetables reduces the risk of breast cancer. Remember, your body is the result of everything you put in your mouth.

If, while reading the list above, you notice that few of these risk factors apply to you, keep in mind that the National Cancer Institute says most people who develop breast cancer have no strong risk factors except for growing older. Breast cancer is not biased—it can strike anyone at any time. Visit the National Cancer Institute Web site at www.cancer.gov for more information.

Diagnostic Mammograms

Your physician orders a diagnostic mammogram when your breast shows abnormal symptoms, including:

- Lumps.

- Thickening.

- Swelling.

- Dimpling.

- Skin irritation.

- Distortion, which is any change from the normal appearance of the breast.

- Retraction, when the nipple is pulled inward.

- Scaly, crusted, red or oozing skin of the nipple and areola (the darker skin around the nipple), which could be an early sign of Paget's disease of the nipple, a rare form of breast cancer that begins in the milk passages (ducts) and spreads to the skin.

- Pain and tenderness of the nipple that do not go away.

If any of these symptoms are present, your physician will order a diagnostic mammogram and, if there's a lump or mass, an ultrasound. No matter what age you are, you should undergo an ultrasound if you have a lump in your breast. Not only women older than 40 get breast cancer; younger women get it, too. Don't think your age will protect you. Remember, my friend Alicia died of the disease at age 27. Your only protection is early detection.

The National Cancer Institute offers a free Breast Cancer Risk Assessment Tool to help you figure out your risk for developing invasive breast cancer, which is cancer that has spread beyond the layer of tissue in which it developed and is growing into surrounding, healthy tissues. It is also called infiltrating cancer. The tool asks questions about your risk factors, such as the number of first-degree relatives with breast cancer, the age at which you had first menstrual period, the number of breast biopsies you've had, your race, and the age at which you had your first baby. Based on your answers, the tool calculates your estimated risk for developing invasive breast cancer over the next five years as well as in your lifetime. To obtain this tool, visit www.cancer.gov/bcrisktool

or contact the Office of Cancer Communications, National Cancer Institute, Building 31, Room 10A03, 31 Center Drive, MSC 2580, Bethesda, Maryland, 20892-2580.

You can visit the National Cancer Institute's home page at www.cancer.gov, and the organization's phone number is (800) 4-CANCER. Another good organization to contact for information is the American Cancer Society, at www.cancer.org or (800) ACS-2345. One more resource to check out is the Web site www.breastcancer.org.

3. Step by Step: An Outline of the Mammogram Process

"I heard they will flatten me like a pancake."

Before Your Mammogram

Screening and diagnostic mammograms are usually done not in your OB-GYN's office but in special mammogram facilities that have their own doctors, called radiologists, who read your films and report back to your doctor. Mammogram facilities must be certified by an FDA-approved accreditation body, which currently includes the departments of health in Arkansas, Iowa, and Texas, as well as the American College of Radiology. For more information, visit www.fda.gov/cdrh/mammography/accreditation.html. The technologists at each facility must also be certified by the state health department and should be licensed by the American Registry of Radiologic Technologists. However, different facilities have different requirements, so a technologist could be licensed by the state health department but not the ARRT.

The Mammography Quality Standards Act is a federal law enforced by the U.S. Food and Drug Administration that is designed to make sure every facility meets quality standards. The MQSA standards apply to the technologists who take the mammograms, the radiologists who study the films, and the medical physicists who test the mammography equipment. Look for the MQSA certificate at your mammography facility and check its expiration date. The certificate ensures that the facility undergoes regular inspections.

One of the most important items you should check for is information about the radiologist who will read your mammogram. Does he or she use an electronic image checker, such as the CAD (computer-aided detection) system? The use of an electronic image checker reduces observational oversights and helps radiologists detect breast cancer early.

If you're seeking extra comfort as well as quality, choose a facility that uses the Woman's

Touch MammoPad®. This FDA-approved cushioning pad is radiolucent, which means it does not interfere with the passage of X-rays and thus has no effect on the quality of X-ray images and does not increase your radiation dose. The MammoPad is a wonderful benefit that I hope every facility will use.

It's important to choose a caring, efficient, high-quality place to have your mammograms. You do not necessarily have to go to the facility your OB-GYN suggests, although you should bring it to your doctor's attention if you have an issue with his or her recommendation. A good way to choose a mammogram facility is by word of mouth. Ask your friends or women in your family for suggestions. Consider going to the facility to make your appointment instead of making it over the phone so you can get a feel for how the place is run and meet some of the staff.

If you have breast implants, mention this to the clinic staff when scheduling your mammogram. They may have to place you in a longer appointment slot, since implants require eight X-ray pictures instead of four.

Your Mammogram Appointment

Remember not to schedule your appointment for any time one week before or during your menstrual cycle, because hormones released during the cycle can cause breasts to feel tender or sore. Caffeine can also cause breasts to become tender and inflamed, especially if you have fibrocystic breast tissue. That means your breasts contain non-cancerous lumpy irregularities (cysts) that can sometimes, but not always, be felt. The cysts increase in size and tenderness before menstruation and recede afterward.

If you consume caffeinated products and you want to know if they make your breasts tender, lie face down on a hard surface for a few seconds and see how it feels. If you feel tenderness in your breasts, evaluate your situation. Ask yourself, "Am I drinking a lot of caffeine? Am I on my period?" Consider giving up caffeine if it does affect your breasts. If you aren't willing to give it up permanently, start cutting back the day you schedule your mammogram appointment so that it will begin filtering out of your system, and don't have any caffeine on the day of your appointment. Coffee, soft drinks, chocolate, some medicines, and non-herbal tea contain caffeine.

On the day of your appointment, don't wear antiperspirant or put talc dusting powder, lotions, or creams on or near your breast area. Some of these products contain aluminum, which can show up on the mammogram and cause you to receive an unnecessary callback. In other words, the facility may call you back to have a second mammogram because the radiologist found suspicious abnormalities while reading your first one. You can, however, wear deodorant that does not contain aluminum. Some facilities provide cleaning wipes in case you do come in wearing antiperspirant.

It doesn't matter what you wear to the appointment, but you will be asked to remove clothing from the waist up, so a two-piece outfit is the most practical.

Keeping your appointment and being on time are very important. If you're late, everyone after you in the appointment schedule will also be late, so if you're not going to arrive on time then call the clinic and let the staff know. After all, how would you feel if you came in on time and then had to wait because other patients were delayed and didn't bother to call? Please be considerate. Remember, if you show up late or on the wrong day, it affects the entire clinic.

In several situations, it may be better to reschedule your appointment—for example, if your period starts or is about to start, or if your breasts feel sore, due to hormone changes or caffeine.

Your Mammogram Records

If you have your previous films, bring them with you to the facility (unless this is your first mammogram, of course). If you do not have your previous films, you should begin trying to locate them as soon as you make your appointment. If you've had a mammogram but can't remember where or when, call the doctor who ordered it and get that information before your next mammogram. You can call the facility where you had the previous mammogram and have the staff mail your films to you or to the facility where your next appointment is scheduled. This way, you will get your mammogram results more quickly. Most importantly, if you are scheduled for a diagnostic mammogram, having your previous mammograms available could be crucial to your diagnosis and possibly to your treatment.

If you can't locate your mammogram records, you will be treated as a first-time patient. This may result in unnecessary callbacks because the radiologist will not have previous mammograms with which to compare your new films. If you move to another city, you can pick up your records and bring them with you. Just remember that once you take custody of those mammogram records, you are responsible for them and you must make sure you know where they are at all times. If the facility requests that you return the records, make sure you do so. If you do not pick them up when you move, make a note of the facility where you had your mammograms so you can locate your records when it's time for your next one.

Your mammogram records are an important part of your medical history, so take extra care when handling them.

The History Sheet

When you arrive at the facility for your appointment, you will be asked to fill out a history sheet. This ensures that the radiologist who reads your mammogram has as much information as possible about your breasts. For example, you should record any previous breast surgeries or scars of any kind on the history sheet. If you've had a biopsy or lumpectomy, the technologist may give you a "scar marker," which is simply a thin, metal wire taped directly onto your scar. Moles should also be marked on the breast, while scars from breast reductions and implants are usually marked on the history sheet only.

The best way to remember your breast history is to keep a record of all mammograms, surgeries (including biopsies), scars, moles, and any other breast-related issues. Consider keeping all this information in a notebook small enough to fit in your purse so you can bring it to your appointment and refer to it while filling out the history sheet. You can call it your "Little Breast Book."

To ensure that you're able to fill out the history sheet thoroughly and accurately, be prepared to answer the following questions (it's a good idea to jot down the necessary information in your Little Breast Book).

What is your name, address, and phone number? Although the doctor who sent you to have the mammogram has this information, it's essential that the mammography clinic also has it because the clinic is responsible for sending you the results of your mammogram and, if needed, calling you back for a follow-up.

Who is your referring physician? The name, address, phone number, and fax number of the doctor who sent you to have the mammogram is necessary to ensure that your results are sent to the correct physician. Multiple doctors in the same area may have the same name, so accurate information is vital.

Have you had a mammogram before? If this is your first mammogram, it will be called your "baseline." It's likely you may get a callback after your baseline mammogram because no previous films exist to help the radiologist judge what is normal or abnormal for your breast tissue. If this is not your first mammogram, the clinic will want to know when and where you had your last one. Some clinics will locate these records for you; others will require that you provide them with that information. Do not answer "no" to this question on the history sheet just because you can't remember where you had your previous mammogram. Simply answer truthfully and say you don't know the location of your records.

Have you had any breast ultrasounds? Your answer to this question will let radiologists know if your breasts have shown any abnormalities in the past and if they should compare any future ultrasounds with previous ones.

Are there any new lumps in your breasts? Mammograms do not detect all breast lumps, which makes this the most important question on the history sheet. Any breast lump in a person of any age—male or female—should undergo an ultrasound.

Are you experiencing pain or tenderness in your breasts? Radiologists use this question to determine if you are experiencing pain because of a cyst that may have formed or become inflamed, which may require antibiotics but not necessarily a biopsy, or if you are experiencing tenderness because of too much caffeine or your menstrual cycle. Localized pain or tenderness may signify an abnormality other than the usual conditions that accompany menstrual cycles, hormone therapy or fibrocystic breasts. Remember, eliminating caffeine can help reduce the discomfort of these conditions.

Nipple discharge? You should record nipple discharge of any kind on the history sheet.

Breast surgeries? Note all trauma and surgeries your breasts have experienced, including mole and beauty-mark removals, tattoos and tattoo removals, biopsies (both needle and excisional), implants, and reductions. This helps reduce unnecessary callbacks.

Implants or breast reductions? Patients who have implants, or who have had their implants removed, will retain internal scars, which can compromise the quality of the mammogram. Patients who have had more than one set of implants must notify the technologist because they will have excessive scarring. If you've had breast reduction or augmentation (implants), tell the technologist before the mammogram. This information is important to ensure you receive the highest-quality films with the fewest retakes.

Have you ever had breast cancer? The radiologist will want to know in which breast you had the cancer, when it was diagnosed, and if you've had a mastectomy, lumpectomy, chemotherapy, radiation, or reconstruction.

Family history of breast cancer? If you answer "yes," you are at risk of developing breast cancer. If you answer "no," you are at risk of developing breast cancer. Remember, breast cancer is not biased—you can develop it whether or not you have a family history. However, if you answer yes, you'll be asked to fill in the ages at which your family members were diagnosed, because the younger they were, the higher your risk.

Do you take any type of hormones? Hormone replacement therapy (HRT), birth-control pills, and thyroid medications are types of hormones. Radiologists want to know about HRT because it can affect the way your breast looks on the mammogram.

Have you had a hysterectomy; if yes, when? Most women who have hysterectomies also undergo HRT, which, again, can cause changes in the breast.

Is there any chance you could be pregnant? Radiation can harm a fetus. If you think you may be pregnant, a pregnancy test will be required before you have your mammogram. Being pregnant will *not* impede your ability to receive medical attention for your breast conditions.

The date of your last menstrual period? This date is important to radiologists because breasts, especially those with fibrocystic tissue, undergo changes throughout the menstrual cycle. For example, some women have benign masses called fibroadenomas that increase in size and tenderness before menstruation and decrease afterward.

What is your reason for having a mammogram? This is an important question because your answer will determine if you receive a screening or diagnostic mammogram. If you are exhibiting no symptoms and simply want to get your annual mammogram, you'll be in the screening category. If you've discovered an abnormality, such as a lump, you will receive a diagnostic mammogram.

It's vital to fill out the history sheet completely and truthfully for two reasons. First, filling out the history sheet inaccurately—failing to mention a previous breast surgery, for instance—can result in an unnecessary callback. That can mean needless worry, stress, cost, and missed hours at work for you. The second reason is because a mammogram is only one of the tools used to detect breast cancer, and the information you supply on the history sheet can determine whether or not you'll need to take advantage of other tools, such as an ultrasound. Incomplete and inaccurate information may prevent the radiologist from recommending the use of other tools, thereby increasing the chance that your breast cancer will remain undiagnosed.

Some women don't fill out the history sheet completely because they think their symptoms are unimportant. However, what you think is nothing may very likely be significant to the radiologist. For example, let's say you've noticed scaliness or subtle dryness around the nipple, but when you go in for your mammogram you don't think it's worth writing down on the history sheet. However, scaliness and dryness may be early symptoms of Paget's disease of the breast, a form of cancer. If you don't write down *every* change in your breast, no matter how insignificant you think it is, your cancer may go undetected until the condition worsens.

Other women may not properly fill out their history sheets because they are frightened or in denial. Recently, a patient came into my clinic for her first mammogram. She checked "no" for all of the questions on the history sheet, including "Are there any new lumps in your breast?" Later, I learned that she had found a lump in her breast several days earlier, which impelled her to have the mammogram. Maybe she subconsciously thought that filling out the history sheet with false information would somehow make her cancer disappear. What she apparently didn't think about was that her decision to check "no" could have been deadly. If she had shown me where she felt the lump, I would have marked the area and, whether or not any abnormality showed on the mammogram, the radiologist would have automatically ordered an ultrasound follow-up. Instead, it was left up to chance. As it happened, the mammogram did show an abnormality, which caused her to return for a follow-up. However, if it had not been evident on the film, the cancer could have gone undetected and spread throughout her body. The decision to lie on the history sheet could have cost that patient her life.

Remember, a mammogram does not catch every incidence of breast cancer, but it is still an essential tool for detecting the disease. It takes all three tools—monthly breast self-exams, annual clinical exams and yearly mammograms—to follow the motto that every woman should memorize: Early detection is your only protection.

During Your Mammogram

When you go into the room where you'll get your mammogram, you'll be asked to put on a gown, which usually opens to the front. It can be a scary time, especially if it's your first mammogram, so you should be in a friendly atmosphere. The technologist should also be friendly. If she walks into the room and tells you it's going to hurt, that's your first clue that you should exercise your rights as a patient and ask for another technologist, or even go so far as asking for the supervisor if necessary.

Your screening mammogram should not be painful. But don't feed the flame and then complain—in other words, if you have fibrocystic breasts, you're on your period and you drink caffeine regularly, it's likely that your breasts will be sore. However, a screening mammogram can still be relatively comfortable even if you've had caffeine and are on your period—if the technologist is made aware of these conditions. Don't be afraid to talk to her. Your technologist should act compassionately toward your breast conditions, even if you have been "feeding the flame." Clinics usually have more than one technologist on staff, so if you don't feel comfortable with the one you have, request another. Do not, however, underestimate the importance of proper breast compression, which I'll talk about later in this chapter.

Once you're in the room, your technologist should explain to you the steps she's going to take.

The standard screening mammogram consists of four pictures. However, the technologist decides how many pictures to take, and the sequence in which to take them, based on each patient's body shape. With a good technologist and a cooperative patient, this should not be an unpleasant process.

The Mammogram Machine

Mammogram machines come in different makes and models, like cars, but they all do the same thing. Look for a "Certification of the Mammography System" in every mammogram room. Facilities are, by law, not allowed to operate these machines without that certification.

The two types of mammogram machines are analog and digital. Analog machines make an actual film picture of your breast, while digital machines computerize the picture so it can be printed to film or CD. Digital mammography is excellent for dense breasts. It also gives the radiologist who reads your mammogram more options to manipulate the image without giving you additional radiation exposure.

For a screening mammogram, the technologist will usually take the standard four pictures, which provide two different views of each breast. Two of the pictures are called cranial-caudal views, which means the machine will compress the breast from top to bottom. The other two are called mediolateral-oblique views, which means the machine will be angled to suit your body's contours. This view may also give the radiologist a look at your lymph nodes, which can be important because irregularities in that area can signify a breast problem. If you feel discomfort during your positioning, talk to the technologist and explain to her what you're feeling. For example, a technologist may inadvertently create pinching skin folds that she can't see, but if you tell her about it, she can adjust your positioning to make your mammogram so much more comfortable. Most technologists are dedicated to their profession and spend hours in training to perfect their positioning techniques so they can provide radiologists with the best mammogram pictures for each patient. Communication between technologists and patients is vital. Remember, you always have the right to end the mammogram and request another technologist if you feel pain and the technologist does nothing to address your concerns.

It usually takes less than 10 minutes to complete the mammogram's X-ray pictures. Augmented or very large breasts may take longer and require more pictures. Augmented breasts require a minimum of eight X-rays instead of the standard four because the radiologist must see the breast tissue around the implant as well as the breast tissue without the implant in the picture. While it is believed that augmented breasts do not have a higher risk of developing cancer, the implant does hide some of your breast tissue, so you should take extra care in doing your breast self-exams. Ask your technologist or doctor for detailed information about self-exams to ensure that you perform them correctly.

What Is Compression?

Compression is the method of placing the breast on the "bucky," a flat surface that contains the X-ray film, and then lowering the compression paddle and applying pressure to the breast. It will feel cold, unless the facility is using the Woman's Touch MammoPad®, which is placed on the bucky. Technologists cannot heat the bucky because warmth spreads bacteria and could damage the equipment. Mammogram machines have various sizes of compression paddles; the size of your breasts will determine which paddle the technologist uses.

Like analog machines, digital machines also compress your breasts, but some manufactures offer "flexible" paddles that conform to your breast, making compression more comfortable. Even with analog machines, however, your technologist should always be considerate of your comfort. Just remember that without proper compression, your mammogram may miss the signs of breast cancer.

If you want to give yourself an idea of what it will feel like to be compressed, take two small hardcover books, place one on top of your bare breast and one underneath to mimic the bucky and paddle, and gently press your breast between them only until the breast feels taut. During a mammogram, you'll want to have the most compression you can tolerate without pain. The more compression you tolerate, the more the tissue spreads and allows the radiologist a clear view of underlying breast tissue. Keep in mind that breast cancer can start very, very small. Undetected and untreated, the cancer will grow into a disease that's very difficult to control. The earlier the detection, the less aggressive your treatment will be.

While undergoing compression, remember that caffeine intake, hormones, and your menstrual cycle all play a part in affecting how your breast will react to compression. Also, the level of compression necessary for a successful mammogram varies from woman to woman.

However, excessive compression is never necessary—there is a difference between tight and painfully tight. You should not feel compression to the point of bruising. Again, your communication and cooperation with the technologist is essential to achieve the right level of compression for you. During a screening mammogram, if the technologist causes you excessive pain to the point of bruising and does not adequately respond to your attempts to communicate with her, report your experience to your state's board of health.

Why Is Compression So Important?

Radiologists cannot read what they cannot see.

A mammogram is awkward. But you should feel that tight pressure when your breast is compressed, for several reasons. First, the more compression you take—without pain—the less radiation your breast receives during the X-ray. After compression is complete, the first sound you'll hear is the machine preparing to make the exposure. During this time the machine measures the thickness of your breast so it can deliver the correct amount of X-ray radiation through your breast onto the film. Decrease the thickness of your breast, and you decrease the amount of radiation.

Second, compression creates clarity. Breasts are a combination of fatty tissue, glandular tissue, ducts, vessels, and veins. Without compression, the radiologist would not be able to see any nuances in your breasts, let alone a possibly cancerous tumor. Everything would be blurred together. Compressing the breast tissue separates the different densities in your breast, allowing the radiologist to accurately read your mammogram.

Third, you need that tight pressure because the more secure your breast is, the less chance it has to move accidentally during the procedure. Motion compromises the mammogram by causing distortion, blurring, and perhaps a false reading—you may look like you have a lump when you don't. The technologist will ask you to hold your breath to prevent motion, as well. Don't try to take in a deep breath like you would for a chest X-ray; just stop breathing for a few moments while the exposure is being made. With digital mammography, holding your breath is not necessary.

No two people have exactly the same type of breast tissue, so women require varying amounts of compression to achieve the same results. The breast tissue of a woman who has breastfed several children will be less dense—and therefore need less compression—than the tissue of a woman who hasn't had children.

Alert the technologist if you feel she is overcompressing you, so she can take steps to address your concerns. Relaxing your chest during compression is extremely important because it allows the technologist to get more breast tissue positioned correctly on the film, thus reducing your discomfort.

Once the exposure is complete, the paddle will automatically release your breast. Don't try to pull away until the release occurs. Keeping your chest wall pressed firmly against the bucky will ensure that you receive the most comfortable compression.

After Your Mammogram

You should not feel bruised or painfully sore after the mammogram. Depending on your breast type and the conditions under which the mammogram was performed—if you were on your period or you consume excessive amounts of caffeine—you can alleviate any minor soreness with over-the-counter pain reliever, such as Tylenol, if needed. I emphasize, however, that with a skilled mammographer, an efficient facility, and your cooperation, a screening mammogram should be painless.

The time it takes to get your results varies among facilities, but the FDA requires that all women who get a mammogram be notified of the results by mail within 30 days, unless the results suggest cancer, in which case patient must be notified as soon as possible, preferably within five business days. By law, a letter with the results must be sent to the patient and to the physician who ordered the mammogram. If you have any questions about your results, discuss them with that physician.

The mammogram results will be labeled with a Breast Imaging and Reporting Data System (BI-RADS) category between 0 and 5:

- Category 0: The findings are incomplete, and additional imaging is needed.

- Category 1: Results are negative, meaning there is nothing on which to comment.

- Category 2: A benign (non-cancerous) condition was found.

- Category 3: The results are probably benign but a follow-up should be performed promptly.

- Category 4: The findings show a suspicious abnormality that may warrant a biopsy.

- Category 5: A malignant tumor is highly likely, and the appropriate action must be taken without delay.

Many patients think that if breast cancer doesn't show up on their mammograms, they don't have the disease. This can be a fatal assumption. As I mentioned before, some lumps won't appear on a mammogram. That's why clinics use a variety of tools, including mammograms, biopsies, and ultrasounds, to help detect breast cancer. Ultrasounds can detect certain abnormalities better than mammograms can—and vice versa—so all lumps should be investigated with an ultrasound. A woman younger than the usual mammogram age of 35 should have an ultrasound for any lump she feels.

Most women don't have mammograms before age 35 because their breast tissue is typically too dense to X-ray without making the film to difficult to read. After age 35, the breast tissue starts to break down into more fatty tissue, which is easier to X-ray. Women who have not yet reached mammogram age should perform breast self-exams every month and have a clinical breast exam every year.

Women sometimes ask why they can't just get an ultrasound instead of a mammogram. An ultrasound, a procedure in which sound waves are bounced off tissue so that the echoes produce a picture, will show lumps that a mammogram won't pick up. However, mammograms pick up microcalcifications, which are tiny deposits of calcium that may or may not be cancerous. The mammogram is a great tool for detecting these microcalcifications, but the ultrasound is the better tool for investigating breast lumps.

Again, mammograms were never designed to detect all breast cancers, but they will detect cancers that you cannot yet feel and that can only be seen on the film. Mammograms can catch breast cancer so early, even in the precancerous stage, that you don't have to lose your breast or have chemotherapy or radiation therapy. For example, the mammogram can detect ductal carcinoma in situ, which occurs in the lining of the milk ducts and has not spread to other parts of the breast or body. That means the cancer is still in the duct and can be removed, possibly without any further treatment.

A ductogram, also known as a galactogram, is another way to detect ductal carcinoma in situ.

Ductograms may also be performed on women who have spontaneous nipple discharge. The idea of the ductogram is more uncomfortable than the actual procedure, in which a tiny catheter is inserted into the nipple so that it can inject dye into the ducts. Then, the technologist takes an X-ray of the dye lining the ducts to determine if cancerous cells are present. The procedure is quick and painless.

Of the estimated 59,390 new cases of ductal carcinoma in situ each year, nearly all of them can be cured if diagnosed early. I tell women every day: Don't be afraid of getting breast cancer. Be afraid of not finding it early.

After you've had a mammogram or an ultrasound, the radiologist will determine if a biopsy is necessary, and if so, which type of biopsy you need. Depending on the outcome of your mammogram or ultrasound, you may undergo one of the three most common outpatient biopsies:

- Fine needle aspiration, in which tissue or fluid is removed with a needle and then examined by a pathologist under a microscope. A pathologist is a doctor who identifies diseases by studying cells and tissues.

- Stereotactic biopsy, which uses a computer and a three-dimensional scanning device to find a tumor and guide its removal so a pathologist can examine it.

- Ultrasound-guided biopsy, which is similartostereotacticbutusesultrasound technology to locate abnormal tissue and guide its removal so a pathologist can examine it. This type of biopsy is usually used for breast lumps, while stereotactic is used to investigate abnormal microcalcifications.

Depending on the biopsy results, you may also undergo an excisional biopsy, a surgical procedure in which an entire area or lump is removed and examined by a pathologist.

Eighty percent of lumps investigated with a biopsy turn out to be benign (non-cancerous) tumors. The most common of these benign conditions are fibrocystic changes, which affect many women. Fibrous breast tissue, mammary glands, and ducts overreact to the normal hormones produced during ovulation, causing fibrous lumps or numerous small cysts (lumpy, fluid-filled sacs or "pockets") to develop in the breasts. These changes are most common in women between the ages of 20 and 50 and are unusual after menopause unless the woman is taking hormones.

Cystic mastitis is the tenderness that occurs at the onset of your period and decreases after your period—this is also a condition, not a disease. Again, it's best not to schedule your mammogram for the week before or during your period. If you have either fibrocystic changes or cystic mastitis, you should avoid caffeine and ask your doctor about taking vitamin E to decrease the tenderness and swelling. Research has reported that the chemical methylxanthines found in coffee, tea, cola, chocolate, and some diet and cold medications seem to promote the growth of fibrocystic lumps. In my professional experience, women who stopped using these products found that their cysts gradually disappeared. These women also reported less discomfort during their mammograms.

Other non-cancerous conditions include fat necrosis, which often develops in response to a bruise or blow to the breast. It most frequently occurs in obese women with very large breasts and can easily be mistaken for breast cancer. These lumps are removed surgically. Again, any lump developing in your breast, at any time, should have an ultrasound to determine if a biopsy is necessary.

Don't fear biopsies; they are one of the first steps toward a cure. While mammograms and ultrasounds are excellent for detecting potential breast cancer, examination by a pathologist is the only way to find out for sure whether or not you have the disease. Think of biopsies like mammograms—a vital tool in saving your life through early detection.

4. Breast Self-Exams

"I just don't know what I'm looking for."

I always ask my patients: "Are you checking your breasts every month?"

I've heard all kinds of answers.

"No."

"Sometimes."

"I don't know what I'm looking for."

"My breasts just feel lumpy all over."

"My breasts are so small, I'd know if something was there."

"My doctor checks them every year."

"I try to, when I think about it."

"My husband checks them."

"My breasts are too big."

"I don't have time."

I can't listen to those excuses without trying to change the attitudes of the women who give them, especially when I consider that many of the tens of thousands of people who will die of breast cancer this year could have been saved with early detection and treatment. The American Cancer Society reports that approximately 212,920 women and 1,720 men will be diagnosed with invasive breast cancer in 2006. Those figures exclude carcinoma in situ of the breast, which accounts for more than 60,000 new cases annually.

Here are a few tips to help you keep a watchful eye over your breast health every day.

- Leave your bra off while putting on your makeup or getting ready in the morning. Get into the habit of watching for changes such as inverting nipples, discoloration, dimpling, peau d'orange (when the skin of your breast becomes swollen and shiny with deep, enlarged pores, like the peel of an orange) or any other change from your normal shape and appearance.

- It's easier to feel lumps when your skin is wet and soapy in the shower. Every time you bathe, make a quick sweep of your breasts with your hands to check for lumps, especially under your arms and around the upper, outer part of your breast, near your armpit, where many breast cancers occur. Don't forget to check the lower, outer quadrant of your breast near your rib cage; the inner, upper, and lower parts near your sternum; and behind the nipple. This is also a good time to do a few breast exercises. For example, put your palms together in front of you, elbows bent so they point toward your left and right, creating a rectangular space between your forearms and your chest. This is also known as the old "I must, I must, I must increase my bust" technique. While you won't increase your breast size, this exercise will benefit your body by increasing blood circulation, and it will strengthen the muscle that supports your breasts, which will make having a mammogram more comfortable.

• While putting on your bra every morning, scan your breasts for any changes in appearance. Try it the next time you're getting dressed. You'll be surprised how this easy, everyday action can promote your breast-health awareness.

Follow these day-to-day tips in addition to, not instead of, your monthly breast self-exam, or BSE. Instructions for performing a BSE are available from your doctor's office and on the Internet. Instead of viewing a BSE as a monthly hassle, you should embrace it as a life-saving tool that you *want* to use, since more breast cancers are found through self-exams than by any other method. How often does a medical practice come along that not only is so successful at keeping you healthy but also can be easily and conveniently done at home? The steps are simple:

1. While lying on your bed, elevate your right shoulder with a pillow or towel. Put your right arm above your head. With your left hand, gently examine your right breast using the pads of your fingers (not your fingertips). Cover the entire breast area with up-and-down or circular motions, from the lymph node area under your arm to behind the nipple and under the breast. Repeat on the other side. Do not squeeze your nipples during the BSE, but do report spontaneous nipple discharge to your physician, especially if it's bloody.

2. In front of a mirror, stand with your arms relaxed by your side and look for any swelling, dimpling, inverting or retracting nipples (when the nipple

appears to be pulled in), and other changes in your breasts. Place a good light off to one side rather than directly above the mirror because side lighting helps to show irregularities.

3. Raise your arms above your head. Then, clasp your hands in front of your forehead while squeezing your palms together to tighten the chest pectoral muscles. Finally, place your palms flat on the sides of your hips and press downward. This highlights bulges, lumps, indentations, dimpling, and any other possible breast changes. During each of these three poses, look for irregularities in your breasts.

For other ways to perform BSEs, consult your doctor's office or the Internet to find a method you like. No matter which method you choose, monthly BSEs are critical in saving your breast and your life.

If you find a lump or other breast change during a self-exam, DO NOT IGNORE IT. Denial can cost you a breast, or even your life. Early detection and treatment increase your chances for survival. In fact, the American Cancer Society reports that the five-year survival rate for people whose breast cancers are treated in the early, localized stages is 96 percent.

Remember to perform the monthly self-exam a week after your menstrual cycle because your breasts go through changes before and during your cycle. If you no longer have a cycle, pick a date that's easy to remember, like the first of the month.

And mothers, teach your daughters. The American Cancer Society recommends that women begin performing BSEs at age 20 as part of a three-part program that also includes mammograms and clinical breast exams. Self-exams should continue even through pregnancy and menopause. My opinion is that if a girl starts performing BSEs when she begins to develop breasts, she'll be firmly in the habit by the time she's 20. It will be as natural to her as wearing a seat belt. Also, a woman should begin getting yearly clinical breast exams at the same time as her first Pap smear, preferably by age 18.

Women with breast implants must be even more diligent in doing their self-exams. While implants do not increase your risk of getting breast cancer, they do make it harder to detect breast cancer because they block out tissue normally seen on a mammogram. That's why Dr. William Ecklund developed the Ecklund method, so women with implants could get more effective mammograms. With this method, the technologist takes twice as many pictures during the mammogram. First, she takes four pictures that include the implants to check for leakage. Then the technologist takes four pictures of the "push-back views," which means she pushes back the implant while positioning your normal breast tissue. This procedure should not be painful and should be done by an experienced technologist. Remember, don't be afraid to ask for a different technologist if you are not comfortable with the one you have.

Even with the Ecklund method, implants still block much of the normal breast tissue during mammograms, which make self-exams and clinical exams all the more important. Don't be afraid to push around the implant to feel your chest wall. You need to check this area every month, while also checking behind your nipples and using your mirror to check for any changes in your breasts.

If we all take advantage of the four safety measures—quick daily checks, monthly BSEs, yearly mammograms after age 40, and yearly breast checks by a doctor—we can successfully combat this cancer. Remember, early detection is our only protection.

5. Men and Breast Cancer

"I was too embarrassed to go to the doctor. Men aren't supposed to get breast cancer."

Early detection is just as important for men as it is for women.

The National Cancer Institute estimates that 2,030 new cases of breast cancer will occur in men in 2007. Men who have female relatives with breast cancer are at higher risk than the general population. Other risk factors include a history of testicular abnormalities, infertility, breast trauma, nipple discharge or nipple bleeding, and a rare genetic disorder called Klinefelter's Syndrome.

Close to a quarter of the men diagnosed with breast cancer are expected to die from it. Men with breast cancer suffer from a lack of public awareness, which may cause some men to ignore early warning symptoms and avoid telling their doctors. This can cause men's breast cancer to be diagnosed at a more advanced stage and perhaps even spread to the lymph nodes. Like women, men should report any changes in their breast conditions, no matter how small, to their doctor. Women can help the men in their lives watch out for breast cancer by passing along the information in this book and making sure that a man who notices an abnormality promptly visits his doctor. Men should not feel embarrassed or uncomfortable if their doctors send them to a breast center to have the abnormality checked out.

A common, benign, but sometimes painful condition called gynecomastia, which causes men's breast tissue to swell under the nipple, can be confused with breast cancer in men. Mammograms can help differentiate the two, but any suspicious mass should be biopsied to rule out cancer.

Men's breast cancer is usually treated the same way as women's. In fact, much of the information in this book applies to both genders, although men do not have milk ducts and therefore cannot be diagnosed with certain conditions, such as ductal carcinoma in situ.

For more information about men and breast cancer, visit the National Cancer Institute's Web site at www.cancer.gov or call its Cancer Information Service at (800) 4-CANCER.

6. How You Can Help

"Everybody says it hurts so badly."

Encourage, Don't Discourage.

Encourage your mother, sisters, friends, and co-workers to get mammograms every year.

Encourage your daughters to practice self-exams regularly as soon as their breasts begin to develop.

Encourage your husbands and sons to be aware of men's risk of breast cancer.

Encourage other women to share positive information about the life-saving capabilities of mammograms.

Encourage everyone you know to maintain a healthy lifestyle and avoid breast-cancer risks such as obesity, lack of exercise, and the intake of unhealthy foods and beverages.

Encourage yourself and the women around you to educate yourselves on the risk factors of breast cancer and the benefits of mammograms, ultrasounds, biopsies, self-exams, and clinical checkups.

Encourage, don't discourage, because what you say and do can make a life-or-death difference to the people you know.

As an example, I'll tell you about my friend Anna.

I've known her for years, and I knew about her strong family history of breast cancer. I encouraged her to get her baseline mammogram at age 35, which she did, and it was normal. But because we lived in different states and I was so busy with my life, I never ask her if she continued getting her mammograms every year or, at the very least, every other year.

As it turned out, Anna didn't get another mammogram until five years later, when she turned 40. I was devastated when she called and told me she was diagnosed with invasive ductal carcinoma.

The cancer had not spread into Anna's lymph nodes, so the plan was to do a lumpectomy and treat her with chemotherapy. After weighing her options, however, Anna decided not to go that route. Because of her strong family history of breast cancer, and the additional risk factor that she'd never had children, she decided to have a double mastectomy with breast reconstruction.

It was not an easy decision, but Anna did not want to chance the cancer coming back. She wanted to go on with the life she enjoys without the worry of a reoccurrence. I am so happy to report that it's been more than a year since they removed the port they placed at the time of her first surgery, and she did not have to endure the chemotherapy after all. The choice she made was best for Anna. She is cancer-free and very happy with her "new" breasts.

But I feel like I let Anna down. It only takes a few seconds to ask your friends if they had their mammograms. Sometimes just a simple reminder is all it takes.

Don't forget to also help yourself. Here's a checklist of the initial steps you should take *today* to begin the journey toward better breast health:

1. Find or buy a small blank notebook to use as a little breast book, and begin compiling all the necessary information, as discussed under *The History Sheet* in Chapter 3.

2. Make an appointment for a mammogram if you don't already have one set up.

3. Do a breast self-exam.

Researchers continuously strive to improve mammography every year, and every year the technology gets better. Mammography has come so far since it was introduced. You may ask, "When are they going to come up with a better way?" I say, "You can't afford to wait for a 'better' way."

Mammography is affordable, effective, and as good as it gets for us right now. Please encourage yourself and others to have mammograms. You, too, could save a life.

Make your promise today!
www.changethestatistic.com

Acknowledgements

To all my patients who inspired me to write this book: Because of you, others will not have to suffer unnecessary pain during screening mammograms. Your experiences serve as inspiration for those who read this book to give mammograms a second chance.

To Dr. Melissa O'Toole, Dr. Debra Butler and Dr. Stephen Rose: My thanks for your continued dedication in detecting breast cancer, for your immense help and support, and for making me a better technologist.

To Dr. Catherine Brandon: Your encouragement helped me believe I could succeed in writing this book. Thank you.

I would like to give special thanks to my editor and friend, Tara Mullee, for all her hard work and devotion in helping me make this book a reality. Her special talent for words has far exceeded my expectations.

I am so thankful to still have with me my mom, Alberta Aydell, and two sisters, Connie and Karen. Connie, thanks for all the cards, letters, and words of encouragement you sent me during the writing process.

My beautiful children, Jennifer and Joshua: You are the bright lights and loves of my life. To my beautiful Jenny for all the sacrifices you made while I wrote this book—thank you for being there through the darkest of times. I am so proud of you and your accomplishments and I love you with all my heart. For the newest lights in my life, I thank my son Josh and his wife Misty for giving me my beautiful grandson, Tristan James, and granddaughters, Madison Claire and Paityn Rose. I love you. My Son, you have made me so proud!

About the Author

I graduated from radiology school in 1987 and have worked as a mammographer for more than two decades. I taught the basics of radiology to fourth-year students at the Louisiana State School of Veterinary Medicine for three years, and I worked in the area of emergency room trauma for five years. I also spent four months training at the M.D. Anderson Cancer Center in Houston, Texas.

My experience in these fields has helped me relate to those who fear breast cancer and the technology that enables us to detect it. I have traveled to many cities working as a mammographer and educating women and men about mammograms, with the hope of creating a more positive reputation for this life-saving process.

It is my hope that after reading this book, you will share the knowledge you've gained, as well as encourage—not discourage—your friends, family, and even strangers to get a mammogram.

YOU could save a life.

Questions and comments are welcome. You can reach me at caydell@yahoo.com.